ACTIVITY IDEAS

For the Budget Minded

by Debra Cassistre

Elder Books

Forest Knolls California

Library of Congress Cataloging in Publication Data
Main entry under title:
Activity Ideas For The Budget Minded
Cassistre, Debra.

Rev. ed. of: *Free Things for Activity Directors.* c. 1987

1. Activities. 2. Aged—Home care.
3. Nursing home care.

LCCN 94-070600
ISBN 0-943873-05-3

Cover and Book Design: Bonnie Fisk-Hayden

Printed in the United States of America

Table of Contents

Introduction

Like most activity directors these days, you are
probably working on a shoestring budget. Even if
you are not yet cashing in coke bottles to supple-
ment your activities allowance, the chances are
you could still use a little more. With that in
mind, *Activity Ideas For The Budget Minded* puts
dozens of creative budget-stretching ideas at
your fingertips. These low or zero-cost activities
will help spice up your program, create variety
and give residents the kind of stimulation and
enjoyment they deserve. Although these activities are mostly geared to older adults, many can
be adapted for use with any group.

CHAPTER 1

Connections

Connections are all important to the activity director. I cannot stress the importance of establishing them enough. Find them, establish them and use them.

In your files you probably have endless connections that you don't even know or realize. Go over them, paying special attention to the former occupations of residents and their immediate families. If Mrs. Smith has a daughter in town who works for an arts and crafts store, you should already be planning to capitalize on this. Discounts, freebies and craft classes may all result from this connection.

Don't feel embarrassed or timid about being an aggressive 'connector.' Does this make you a user? Don't be ridiculous! You are doing this, not for yourself, but to enrich the lives of your residents in every way possible. You are not a "con-artist." You are a calculating recruiter.

Now that that's out of the way, I'll leave the investigative work to you. Remember, families of residents are your best bet. Find out their occupations, interests and hobbies if you can. (Of course, you can!) If a family member, resident or employee donates yarn for crafts, for example, be sure to show your appreciation in your monthly newsletter, as well as in person. In print you could say "A great round of applause goes to Mrs. Johnston (Mary's daughter) for all the beautiful yarn she donated. We can always use yarn in our crafts department."

Since your newsletter circulates among family and staff, others will read it and get the message—*"we want and need donations."*

For a more specific request (or just in case no one actually donated anything!) it wouldn't be the worst thing in the world to print a slight error. For example, *"Many thanks to the Wilkens family for donating the candy served at our party. It was very sweet and as you know, everyone loves candy."*

Never mind the Wilkens family. (What Wilkens family?). Others will get the hint. Sweets should be forthcoming!

What Can You Get from Connections?

FLOWERS FOR ALL OCCASIONS

If you do a lot of business with a particular florist, ask them for floral arranging demonstrations from time to time. Approach them about donating birthday corsages for your birthday gals each month. They may even let you have the 'extra' flowers which they can't use because of discoloration, broken stems or missing petals. Perhaps they could fashion some little corsages out of these unwanted leftovers each month?

Hopefully, these good hearted folks will comply and make your ladies so very happy. Take photos of the proud birthday people wearing their corsages and include the pictures in your initial thank-you letter for display at the flower shop.

Birthday Greetings

You don't need connections with the President of the United States to get him to send special birthday greetings to your residents. Just write to his office and tell him how many birthday greetings you need for each month. Although the President will not go as far as licking the envelopes himself, you will get a bulk supply. You can hand out the greetings at your monthly birthday celebration.

Write:

Greetings Office
Office of the President
The White House
Washington D.C.

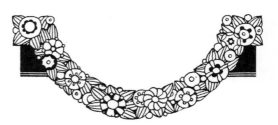

Decorations

You can obtain seasonal and holiday decorations by approaching a local grocery store chain. Most large chains have very acceptable, even innovative, decorations supplied by corporate offices. They are sometimes used as decorative cardboard backgrounds behind various displays and are disposed of after use. Suppliers would happily donate them to your facility just for the asking.

Supplies

Large supermarket chains may also be willing to donate candy and supplies for your cooking class. The stores you frequent most will hold your best chance. Sometimes you can work things out with store managers personally. If not, don't give up! Try writing to the marketing or public relations office with your requests. They can be quite generous at times. Managers will gladly tell you where to address your inquiries. Other good sources for prizes and decorations are card stores, large department stores and drug stores.

PRIZES AND GIFTS

Prizes and gifts can be found all over, but you may have to turn over a few rocks to get them. Avon representatives often have samples of hand lotion, perfume and body oil on hand. If you find a cooperative Avon lady, perhaps she can come and do a make-up demonstration for residents and staff. Help her get orders and she will help you with free samples. The Avon company may also help with leftovers from discontinued merchandise.

Write:

Avon
5000 City Line Road
Newport News VA 23630

CHAPTER 2

Volunteers

A good volunteer program will greatly enhance the activities department. Undoubtedly, you already know this, but still, let me repeat these words to the wise. *Cherish your volunteers, treat them with the utmost respect and seize every available opportunity to praise them (sincerely we hope!) because they are a blessing.*

When you go about recruiting volunteers, be sure to have specific jobs in mind. This will enable you to structure your volunteer program more efficiently. Following is a list of roles they may be able to fulfill.

Crafts assistant
Religious leader (Sunday worship services,
   spiritual healings)
Chaperone
Dancers (great way to liven up a party)
Exercise instructor
Fund raiser
Transportation assistant
Sewing instructor

Group discussion leader
Letter writer
Music specialist
Historian
Party coordinator
Bible study helper
Hymn sing-a-longs
Game night coordinator
Bible Trivia leader
Visiting night assistant
Vespers services assistant

Finding Volunteers

There are many people in the community who would enjoy spending some free time with elderly folks. Since they may not approach you, make it your business to find them. The process is not unlike hunting for treasure! Here are some places to look:

LOCAL CHURCHES

Please don't tell me you haven't already tapped this valuable resource. Churches are just brimming with good folks who feel it is their mission to share their love and render assistance to those in need. (I'd say we definitely qualify there!). Using guidelines set by your administrator, put the volunteers' many talents to good use.

Find out how many different groups there are within the church. For example, there may be a ladies auxiliary; an altar guild; a youth group as well as a junior choir. It's likely that each group will have a penchant for a specific project, so try to match them accordingly. Even if your volunteer group is a religious one, they can deviate from strictly church activities and take part in any of the activities described in this book. Establish a regular meeting time, for example, the first Tuesday of every month at 2:00 p.m, that is convenient for both volunteers and your charges.

ELEMENTARY, JUNIOR HIGH AND HIGH SCHOOLS

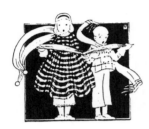

Local schools may be one of your best resources. School bands and choruses often put on terrific shows, some with artistic choreography as well. Older folks show great appreciation for talented youngsters and kids welcome the opportunity to perform for an audience.

SCHOOL CLUBS

Find out about the school's various clubs. Perhaps members from the school's chess club can meet with chess players at your facility on a regular basis? Get the debating club to put on a debate for you. Better yet, try to involve residents. Once you have a list of school clubs, more ideas will come instantly. Think of what

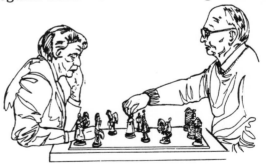

they could do for you and hopefully themselves.

GIRL/BOY SCOUTS

Don't overlook the Girl and Boy Scout clubs in your search for volunteers. These clubs often take on community projects to earn pins and badges. Craft activities such as making decorations are often popular.

GARDEN CLUBS

Invite a green thumb enthusiast to come and conduct a basic gardening class, letting residents plant for themselves. It's therapeutic to watch things grow! Try it.

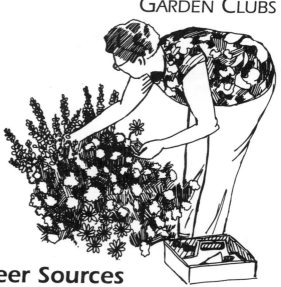

Other Volunteer Sources

Retired Senior Volunteer Program (RSVP)
Gray Panthers
Council on Aging
Golden Age Club
American Association of Retired Persons (AARP)
Local Women's Club
Big Brothers/Sisters
SPCA

Don't forget to ask families and friends of residents to volunteer. They will often get involved for the asking. Remember to have specific jobs lined up.

Good luck!

Volunteer Activities

CHURCH VISITS

Older adults often enjoy visits to church. Once you get involved with church groups, they will probably invite you to attend church on Sunday. If you have transportation and assistance, this activity is sure to be enjoyable for selected residents.

COUPON CLIPPING

Residents who still have use of their hands will enjoy clipping coupons. They can work together in small or large groups. Serve coffee or tea as they clip away. An alert resident can sort the coupons into various categories such as coupon organizers suggest: dairy, meat, frozen foods, paper products, cleaning supplies, etc. A volunteer can help supervise. If employees use the coupons on a regular basis, residents will be encouraged to participate as they will recognize a need for this time-passing activity.

LETTER-WRITING SESSIONS

Schedule regular letter-writing sessions so that your residents mail does not go un-responded to. Volunteers can work with individual residents or in a group setting.

ENVELOPE STUFFING

Envelope stuffing for a charitable organization can be a fun and most useful (and sometimes even profitable) venture. The supervisor of the 'stuffing session' should contact the charity well in advance. Most have annual mail-outs. Other contacts would include anyone who uses direct mail. If necessary, modify the requirements of this activity to meet the abilities of your group.

BEDSIDE VISITS

Have a few volunteers on hand to make bedside visits to residents. They can bring along something to share such as a collection of stamps, a book to read or photographs. Suggest they bring an interesting magazine with colorful pictures to read with the resident.

PUPPETMASTER

If any of your volunteers have a way with puppets, put this skill to good use. Buy simple hand puppets and have the volunteer visit residents wearing these. Hand puppets are wonderful ice-breakers and conversation starters.

SHOW AND TELL

Volunteers can lead special show and tell sessions. They can invite residents to bring something they cherish along to the group and tell group members about it. It might be a photo, jewelry, postcard or a letter. This activity is good for confused residents as the object helps keep their attention focused. It is also a good conversation starter.

RHYTHM BAND

Encourage a volunteer to start a rhythm band. You can buy rhythm band instruments inexpensively or better still, make your own. No special skills are required to join the band.

WALKING

Walking is a healthy activity which should be promoted in every facility. Perhaps a volunteer could start a walking club. Members could walk a little further each day. Indoor walking is pleasurable, but when the weather is fine, make sure residents have an opportunity to go outdoors.

CHAPTER 3

Intergenerational Activities

Make sure that your activities program has an intergenerational component. When children and older adults are together, a special magic is created that cannot be duplicated. Intergenerational activities are especially important for those residents who have no grandchildren or grandnephews and nieces. Children bring joy, love and lightheartedness to their lives and in turn, the children receive undivided attention, quiet time and some of the wisdom of age.

Finding children to take part in the program is not generally difficult. Children of all ages can participate—from preschool through the high school years. Your best contacts for children are local day care centers, junior and high schools as well as summer school programs and churches. Don't overlook one of your best sources: the children of staff members and volunteers.

Adopt-A-Grandparent

The 'adopt-a-grandparent' program is one of the most popular intergenerational activities. Children visit the facility on a regular basis and each child 'adopts' a particular resident. This type of program is not difficult to implement and the rewards are many. The resident gets to spend quality time with a child and experiences the pleasure of a close friendship and regular visits. The child has an opportunity to be listened to and to share important happenings.

Most facilities now have successful 'adopt-a-grandparent' programs in motion. You can spice up the program with special little touches. One favorite activity is to hold a mock adoption ceremony for your adopted little ones. Set up your room like a court room. The "judge" who officiated the ceremony at our facility wore a black robe (a priest's robe borrowed by an employee) and pounded his gavel every time he wanted his court to come to order.

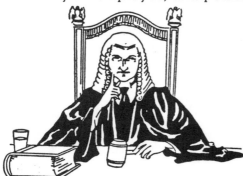

Borrow an American flag, make a nameplate and place it by the judge's bench. The children can stand and recite some well-rehearsed line such as "We the children of Mayberry school promise to give love and affection to our newly-adopted grandparents from Stonegrove facility on the 1st Tuesday of every month." Residents can reciprocate with their own prepared statement. The judge can pound his gavel again and make it official. The more you elaborate on this one, the better. Perhaps the Clerk of the Court can introduce his honor? Alert the local TV stations and newspaper. What a lovely human-interest story.

Baby Day

This activity is fun, but you will have to find the babies first. You could contact a local church with a large congregation and advertise your event there. If you have connections, the event is sure to be well promoted. Schedule visits on a Saturday morning or Sunday afternoon if possible so that working mothers can attend. Have a definite itinerary in mind. Perhaps each parent could introduce their baby

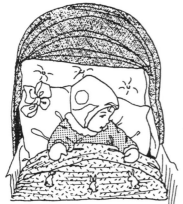

and state their age. Allow for some visiting time and picture-taking if parents do not object.

Stage a diaper derby if you can get the babies to cooperate. Put clean blankets on the floor with babies on one end, parents on the other. Pin large-print first name tags on the backs of their diapers. Have parents call their little ones and the race begins. These tiny competitors will soon have everyone in stitches.

Have your craft class make award ribbons for all who enter the derby. Make up as many categories as you can and award several prizes. For example; the baby with the most hair; the biggest baby; the baby with the loudest cry; the most congenial baby. Parents will treasure the prize ribbons as reminders of your very special event. Try for some publicity on this activity as it's such an attention-getter.

Fashion Show

A youth group in our area was enterprising enough to put on an antique fashion show by borrowing old clothes from a local antique clothes dealer. The teens modeled clothes which residents remembered wearing in their youth. The show was a smashing hit and has since become an annual event. There are many variations on the fashion show theme worth trying. Here are some ideas:

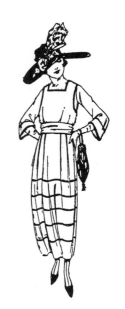

Back to School fashions
Clothes from the 20's, 30's or 40's
Prom Night fashions
Halloween or Easter fashions

NOSTALGIA

Another great activity to share with a youth group is nostalgia night. Have your residents bring old pictures of themselves — the younger the better. Ask teenagers to do the same. This is a wonderful ice-breaker and really sparks conversation.

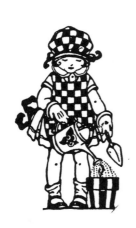

BUBBLE-BLOWING CONTEST

How about a Bubble-Blowing Contest? Line children up in chairs wearing large-print name tags. Provide an ample supply of bubble gum and they'll take it from there. Gag gifts or maybe even bookmarks made by residents can be awarded to round out the event. This is great fun for everyone.

EASTER FUN

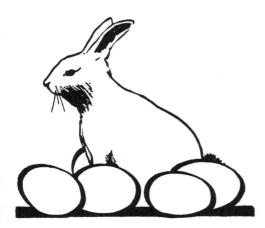

Have residents dye Easter eggs in a variety of colors and invite a local preschool for an Easter egg hunt. Make baskets out of strawberry baskets and ribbons and use pipe cleaners for handles. Have this activity outside in a patio area.

CHARADES

Charades make a cheerful intergenerational activity. Each person in the group acts out the movements while folks guess. Be sure to stand by and offer cues and prompts as needed. If the love is there, it can be considered a mission accomplished.

PEN-PAL CORRESPONDENCE

Encourage a local class to visit your facility and meet with individual residents. Each child can select a resident that he or she would like to correspond with. Schedule regular letter-writing sessions with your residents and have an appointed time (for example, every other Tuesday) for delivery of letters to the school. The children can then reciprocate with letters, pictures, photos or poems. This simple process can evolve into a deep friendship which may last for years.

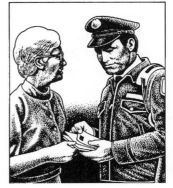

CHAPTER 4

Entertainment on a Shoestring

Dance

Be creative in generating entertainment ideas for residents. Tap local resources. Go through the phone book and call local dance schools. They will often put on wonderful shows for a small donation. Most dance studios schedule a public performance or recital annually. If your facility has adequate space to accommodate the dance troupe, why not offer to let them rehearse there? You may wish to extend this rehearsal invitation to other local groups and bands. In essence, you will be doing a community service by letting these groups "entertain" you at rehearsal.

Choir

Contact public and private schools. Ask to speak with the band or choral director. You will find that many will be glad to perform for your cause. Try to set this up on a regular basis.

If rules permit, have some sort of "inspirational" entertain-

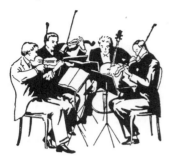

ment once a month. It's usually free and not too hard to find. You may wish to inquire about the adult choir and junior choir. Some churches have handbell choirs that will perform for the asking. Many churches have "outreach" programs where they seek involvement in a community project.

Variety Is The Spice of Life

If you have a regular pianist, try to vary the theme of the performance for the benefit of the activities calendar and newsletter. **The Jill Taylor Show** sounds better that just putting J.T. on the calendar. If someone comes to play piano, dream up interesting ways to bill this event. Old Time Entertainment? Songs of Yesteryear? Old Fashioned Sing-A-Long?

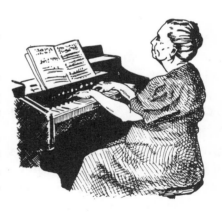

Program themes should be changed regularly to add variety. The person who comes one month for the sing-a-long might next month do a Broadway tune spectacular or hymn sing-a-long. This idea is easily adaptable for any holiday or special occasion theme. For example:

Love Songs for Valentine's Day
Christmas carol sing-a-long

Famous Irish/Scottish folksongs
Songs of summer or winter
Patriotic sing-a-long (4th of July)
German (Octoberfest)
Exaggerate!

Parties

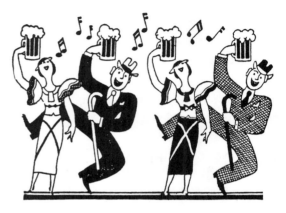

Parties are wonderful entertainment for older adults since they represent a shift from the mundane day-to-day routine. Residents can help plan the event and decide on the time and location. You can make a party at lunchtime by simply having the meal outdoors for a change and bringing along a volunteer who happens to be a wonderful singer.

Exhibits and Displays

Invite a local artist to display some of her paintings in your facility. Call the newspaper or a local radio show and get some publicity for the exhibition. The sight of beautiful paintings adorning the walls will elevate the spirits and bring a little joy and beauty into the lives of residents.

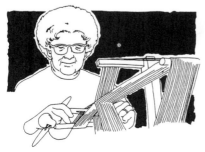

Demonstrations

Invite guests to the facility to share their art or trade with residents. Invite potters, jewelry makers, weavers and photographers in to give a demonstra-

18

tion. A dog-obedience demonstration makes for a fun and interesting activity—especially when held out of doors on a pleasant Summer day. If you can find a juggler, magician or balloon man to come to the facility, then you're really in business!

The Big Bands

Residents will enjoy listening again to the sounds of the Big Band Era—Benny Goodman, Woody Herman, Artie Shaw, Count Basie, Duke Ellington and Tommy Dorsey. The tunes and songs help trigger memories of special moments and events. The Big Band music is now available in a collection of 4 audio tapes called *Big Band Gold*.

The Social Hour

Gather a small group of residents around the table. Serve some nice refreshments and have magazines available as well as a selection of table games. Have some quiet music playing in the background. Let this be a time for residents to mingle, socialize and get to know each other in a small and intimate setting.

Theater

Invite a local theater group to stage a short performance in the facility. Establish a good rapport and they might come back with each new production! The performance might inspire residents to stage their own play which you can direct. There are many good scripts available for older adults.

Bazaar

Hold an occasional bazaar to display and sell products made by residents. This is a real esteem-builder and brings out the hidden talents of facility members. It's also a good fund raising idea. Proceeds from sales can go towards buying new supplies and resources for the activity department.

Cake Baking Contest

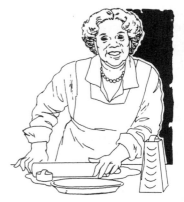

Expect a great turnout for this event! The employees bake cakes (or pies) and residents judge the winners. Offer a $50 bill to the one who bakes the winning cake (use counterfeit money, like the oversize gag money found in gum machines). Applaud all employees for their camaraderie. The official judges can discuss their choice with each participant, and the cake with the most votes wins. Not a half-baked idea!

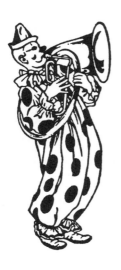

Talent Show

Stage a talent show featuring staff and residents. Have singers and a piano player as well as a clown and any other acts you can dream up. Give a small prize to each performer. This activity is very entertaining and brings out the hidden talents and abilities of facility members.

Outdoor Activities

Outdoor activities provide wonderful entertainment, and many varieties are possible. Outdoor meals including breakfast, lunch or dinner add a special touch to dining. Outdoor movies are wonderful. An outdoor wine & cheese or cocktail party add an extra special touch. Everything from Spelling Bees to an exercise class can take place out of doors. Not all of these ideas will work every time but your efforts will certainly be applauded. So spice up your activities program—with a breath of fresh air!

Historical Programs

Programs depicting historical events which occurred during the residents' youth or middle years will delight. Programs which focus on Abe Lincoln, the World Wars and Franklin D. Roosevelt are usually a hit.

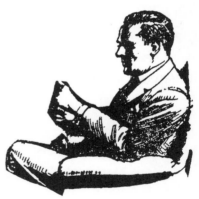

One popular program idea worth trying is "Our City", a historical program about the city in which you live. You might have to dig for material. Invite someone from the city's historical society to give a presentation. If that doesn't gel, try the public library. It is chock full of resource materials including visual aids.

Movies and Films

If you are currently paying for films, consider this information. You can order free 16mm or VHS films from **The Modern Talking Picture Service**. The only thing you have to pay is return postage. They have a large variety of films to suit your viewing pleasure. Subject codes include travel and Geography, vocational guidance, business, sports, safety, homemaking, science and nature as well as many others too numerous to name here.

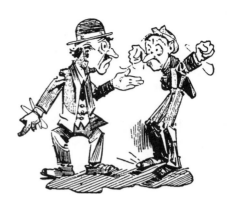

Take advantage of this wonderful free service and have a film festival. Show three short films (15 minutes) back to back in the same day. Serve popcorn!

Send for a free catalog to:

The Modern Talking Picture Service
5000 Park Street North
St. Petersburg FL 33709

CHAPTER 5

Guest Speakers

Guest speakers offer stimulation and enjoyment and bring new energy to the facility. Try to find speakers to match the interests of individual residents. For example, if you have residents interested in quilt making, weaving or writing, locate people who are skilled in these areas in the community. There are so many possible sources for guest speakers that you may decide to feature one every month.

Where To Find Guest Speakers

LOCAL COLLEGES

Colleges often have lists of speakers available for different educational programs. Ask your community college to send you a list of speakers, if one is available. Share the list with residents and let them decide on a guest speaker to invite.

FIRE DEPARTMENT

The fire department will usually send a speaker for the asking. The program should be very interesting and informative. The guest speaker may want to show residents the proper way to use a fire extinguisher and will allow them to actually put out a small fire set outside. I'll leave that option to you...!

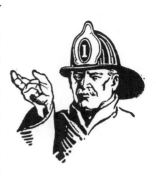

POLICE DEPARTMENT

Call your local police department and ask if a uniformed policeman (visual addition to the program) will give a talk in your facility. He might consider speaking on crime prevention and the elderly or another related topic. You might also invite him to talk to residents about his job and the kinds of challenges a 'typical' working day presents. He or she might also be willing to bring a police dog along.

SPCA

Ask your local SPCA to send a speaker along to talk about their work. They could bring an animal or slides along to enliven the presentation. Residents might be interested in learning about animal care and about ways in which they can help the work of the SPCA.

HEALTH CENTER

Invite a masseuse from a local health center to give a talk on the benefits of massage. She may be willing to give a demonstration. An ideal way to round off this session would be to have residents give hand or back massages to each other, under the skillful guidance of the masseuse.

MEDITATION CENTER/ASHRAM

Meditation is gaining popularity as an effective stress-reducing and health-enhancing technique. Most towns and cities now have several centers which offer regular meditation sessions. Invite a meditation teacher to your facility to explain the benefits of this technique and invite her to lead your group into this blissful and elusive state.

HOSPITALS

Hospitals usually maintain a well-staffed community relations department and have many qualified guest speakers on hand who concentrate on public education. Some health related topics you may inquire about are:

Alzheimer's Disease
High Blood Pressure
Stroke Rehabilitation
Memory Techniques After Illness
Diabetes
Medical advances, such as heart surgery, laser surgery or cancer research

Speakers from these organizations usually bring with them some very interesting educational films.

MARCH OF DIMES

Invite a representative from the **March of Dimes** to make a presentation. Residents will remember well the **March of Dimes'** successful fight against polio during Franklin D. Roosevelt's days. Most will marvel at the amazing medical advances this organization has made in the prevention of birth defects.

PODIATRIST

Do you have a house Podiatrist that regularly visits your facility? What a wonderful way for new residents to become acquainted. Ask him to speak on foot-related problems that elderly citizens might have experienced or total foot care for older adults.

TRAVEL AGENT

If you can find a travel agent who is just starting out, he or she may want to have your business and volunteer to visit your facility. Perhaps you could arrange a short visual presentation such as a film or slide show. Make it a travelogue!

FOOT REFLEXOLOGIST

Invite a reflexologist in to give a demonstration of this unique and therapeutic foot massage. Still a relatively new approach, reflexology is gaining in popularity and residents will be amazed to learn about and experience its effects.

MUSIC CLUBS

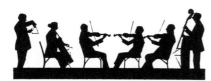

Invite a local music group to perform for residents and to talk about their instruments. This session will be particularly interesting if ethnic musicians and instruments are included. Give residents an opportunity to hold the instruments and if possible, let them experiment.

LOCAL POLITICIANS

Politicians are always willing to visit around election time. Try to persuade them to drop in at other times of the year too. It can be a real morale booster for residents to feel that they are important enough to take up a busy politician's time. Check with administration before you decide which politicians to invite!

POETRY SOCIETY

Invite a well-know local poet to come and talk about the art of writing poetry. Perhaps she will be able to inspire residents to write poetry as a way of expressing thoughts and feelings. Ask her to give a poetry reading.

PHOTOGRAPHER

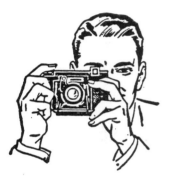

Invite a local photographer to come and talk about all the elements involved in taking a good picture. He can also show residents how a camera works and demonstrate some of his work.

CHIROPRACTIC

Chiropracty is a profession gaining in popularity, and one which may not be familiar to many residents. Give them an opportunity to learn about this interesting new medical approach by inviting a chiropractor to make a presentation. What is the science of chiropractic? How does it help millions each year?

PUBLISHING HOUSE

Invite a local publisher to the facility to talk about the steps involved in publishing a book. Ask her to bring samples of published works and to talk about how the publishing industry has changed since the advent of desktop publishing.

Other good sources to check for guest speakers:

The Health Department
The Kidney Foundation
Center for Hearing Impaired
Center for the Blind
Heart Association
Red Cross
Arthritis Foundation
American Cancer Society
Lung Association
Acupuncture/Acupressure
Audubon Society or Bird Sanctuary
Science Center
Local Meteorologist
Ophthalmologist/Optometrist

With all these resources at hand, you can easily have regular guest speakers. Don't forget to invite family and friends of the facility to speak on selected topics.

CHAPTER 6

Games We Love

There are a wealth of games available for residents of all functional levels. Avoid using board games for reasons an activity director can surely understand. Board games are confusing to some and exclude visually impaired players. Besides which, it takes too much time to use a board game with large numbers of players. Following are games which most groups find enjoyable.

Trivia

Playing trivia in long-term care facilities is a great crowd pleaser and a permanent no-cost addition to your activities calendar. Providing attainable challenges to willing participants also ignites the spirit of old fashioned competition.

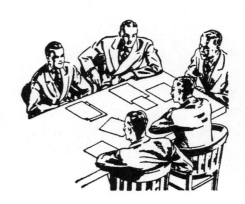

If you have six or more players, divide them into teams. Line chairs up at both sides of a long table and place the officiator at the head. Give peppermint candies out to individual players to signify points earned. Each candy represents one point for a correct answer. At the end of the game, count to see who has the most candy and determine your winner. Team scores can be tallied on paper. Candy or other goodies can be awarded to the winning team. You will soon learn that prizes mean so little in this game because it is simply so much fun.

The Secret of Success

The secret to staging a successful trivia match is to have on hand plenty of suitable questions for elderly contestants. This is crucial to the popularity of the game. For example, if confronted with a series of questions that only a nuclear physicist could answer, residents will withdraw and feel ill-informed, not to mention bored. The most popular trivia games on the market contain far too many questions that are not relevant to the lives of the elderly and their intellectual realm of thought. Not to insult their intelligence, they should be presented with challenges—reasonable ones. Follow this advice and you will see their eyes sparkle with pride as more and more correct answers are given. Proper quiz material will make this game a success and keep them coming back again and again.

So, what is proper quiz material? I repeat. Questions that are relevant to the lives and realm of thought of older adults. You might try taking time before each game to pick out questions of particular appeal. Try using Junior editions of the usual trivia games. Some of these questions will take residents back to childhood as many are based on popular nursery rhymes and major events in history.

You may soon feel a need for more challenging questions.

That's great as any of the popular games or trivia booklets should satisfy that growth potential.

SAMPLE TRIVIA QUESTIONS

1. Name the theater where President Lincoln was assassinated. (Ford)
2. Who spoke of "The New Deal?" (F.D.R.)
3. What were the first names of The Wright Brothers? (Orville and Wilbur)

Remember to accommodate your contestants and good luck!

Other games

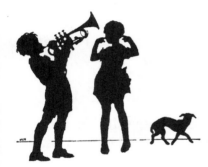

NAME THAT TUNE

It's always nice to have an accordionist or pianist officiate during Name That Tune. If you haven't got one available, record albums will suffice. Play the beginning (or middle or end) of the song until someone raises their hand. Handicapped participants can ring bells for attention.

WHAT'S MY LINE?

This activity takes a little more organizing on your part, but has proven to spark memory in a most interesting way. Prepare sample questions in advance and hand several copies out at the event.

For example:

Did you need special training/studies to do this job?

Did you work indoors?

Did you work outdoors?

Did you wear a uniform?

Did you provide a service?

Did you work with your hands?

Did you stand for long hours?

Did you sit for long hours?

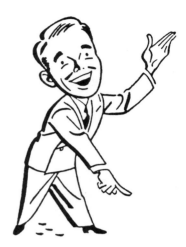

Like the TV game rules, contestants may answer only 'yes' or 'no' questions. You take charge as a referee helping the game along ever so slightly. This event will generate new friendships among residents with common interests and occupations. Everyone likes to talk about the good old days. Since work is like flour in cake—the main structure of our lives—this activity breeds more material to reminisce about.

NAME-O-BINGO

No one has to tell us about bingo. They love it. We hate it. (Sometimes!) But here's a new twist guaranteed to make folks go "out on a limb" and talk to fellow residents.

Name-O-Bingo requires 'home-made' blank cards which instead of BINGO, carry NAME-O across the top. The squares are blank and residents must approach other residents to sign a square (one square only). When the sheets are full of names, the activity director draws at random the names of residents living in the facility. The rest is the same. I always find that a cash prize ($2 bill) usually inspires the most participation. It certainly encourages residents to talk to one another! Another day have them fill in their own lucky numbers instead of names.

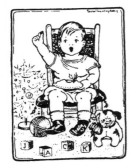

WHO'S WHO

Ask residents to submit baby pictures of themselves for display on a large bulletin board. Exclude their names and have everyone identify the faces.

LAS VEGAS DAY

This gambling game will take a little organizing on your part, but is sure to produce favorable results. You will need volunteers to operate and officiate the games. Award each resident initially with 25 chips so that everyone can participate. Stress that no actual money is necessary so the game cannot be mistaken for "real gambling." Volunteers 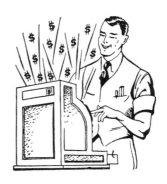 can help deal poker and blackjack and spin the roulette wheel. They can also award chips to winners. At the end of the day, allow the winners to cash in chips for real prizes. Decide on what the chips are worth, for example, 30 chips for a free hairdo.

LET'S MAKE A DEAL

It won't be too difficult to create your own version of the favorite TV game. Wrap several large (and small) boxes with brightly colored paper. Aluminum foil can also be used. Add ribbons and bows, but make sure bottoms of boxes are open so you can add new prizes. You must be able to replenish your supply of deals in private so that residents cannot possibly know what they are trading for. Perhaps you can use an adjoining room or go behind a curtain. Invite residents to bring articles to trade—the funnier the better. (A bedpan, a piece of crumpled paper?) Number boxes and trade away. You should have nice prizes as well as humorous ones. If you want everyone to go crazy with laughter, use an old bra or corset as a gag. Hopefully, a man will win it. Give him a chance to trade it in. The Salvation Army or Goodwill will give you many ideas for prizes. Go prize hunting!

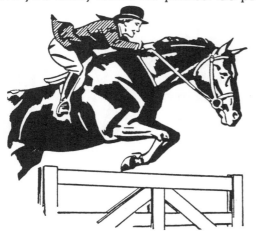

Horse Races

This exciting action game is worth trying, but I'll leave the financial arrangement of the horse track up to you. Cut 5 or 6 figures of horses from cardboard and staple them to poles that have stands on the bottom. The horse, affixed to the pole (or old broomstick) must be able to stand alone. Add different color saddles to each horse (the horses can be different colors as well) with numbers. Make up zany names for them. Use bingo balls (B) 11-15, (I) 21-25, (N) 31-35, (N) 41-45, (G) 51-55 and if you have a sixth horse (O) 61-65. Paying no attention to the letters, let each first digit signify which horse to move and the second number indicate how many spaces to move it. For example, if you draw G 54, that would mean horse #5 would move 4 spaces. Designate spaces on the floor with masking tape. Crown the winner of each race with a wreath of red roses. Make it out of old cardboard cut into a horseshoe shape and add leftover red Christmas bows. Attach a blue ribbon to the wreath. You can also serve traditional mint juleps at this event.

I'll leave it to you to figure out the betting end of this game. Scrap paper tickets could be made up with, for example, 1-5 on it, meaning first race, fifth horse. Playing with pennies would make it even more fun, but be careful. Anyone remember the Largo 8? Gambling is illegal and some folks will go to any lengths (even ridiculous ones) to enforce their beliefs.

THE PRICE IS RIGHT

Another TV game show easily adaptable for our special contestants is **The Price is Right**. Have prizes of all sizes and shapes on hand (ask families for donations). You can go by the original price (if it is marked) or, using your knowledge of the current price market, mark your own. Sit participants (picked from your "studio audience") at a table in full view of the (hopefully) curious spectators. Introduce one product at a time and follow with an elaborate description. Next, ask residents to guess the actual retail value (on a small piece of paper) of the item, without going over the price. The closest guess (without going over) wins, 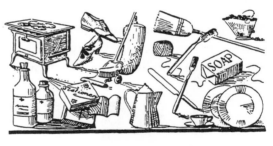 just like on TV. Be sure to encourage your audience to applaud. After a contestant has won two prizes, ask them to retire to their seat and invite someone else to take his/her place.

SPELLING BEE

Spelling Bee is a familiar and popular game. Keep in mind not to make it too difficult or you will frustrate the players. As a variation, divide residents into teams and ask them to define the words instead of spelling them. (A dictionary can be used as a prize.)

CHAPTER 7

Easy Cooking Projects

Cooking together provides an opportunity for relaxed sharing. Residents·have a chance to exchange special recipes as well as memories of favorite foods. Since cooking was a necessary and favored activity in older times, it will evoke memories of the kitchen, of growing up and of mother's cooking.

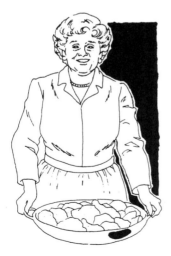

cooking. Encourage your residents to reminisce as they cook.

Here are a few recipes that are safe, fun and good exercise for arthritic hands and fingers. Very little actual cooking is involved. These activities also make excellent fun(d) raising projects.

TRUFFLES

A single recipe makes 36 truffles or 1½ lbs.

Ingredients

1 12 oz. pkg. semi-sweet chocolate pieces
¾ cup sweetened condensed milk
1 tsp. vanilla extract
⅛ tsp. salt

For garnish use any of the following:

½ cup cocoa *or*
1 cup flaked coconut *or*
chopped nuts *or* rice crispies
or powdered sugar *or*
use your imagination

Directions

1. In double boiler over hot, but not boiling water (or in heavy 2 qt. saucepan over low heat), melt chocolate pieces. Stir in condensed milk, vanilla and salt until well mixed. If there is a problem with letting residents use the stove, this part of the project can be done by the activities director.

2. Refrigerate mixture about 45 minutes or until easy to shape.

3. With buttered hands, shape mixture into 1 inch balls. Roll balls in your choice of garnish.

SHORT-CUT DONUTS

Using canned biscuits and old plastic pill bottles as donut holers, separate biscuits and flatten sightly with palm. The plastic medicine container works as an excellent donut holer. Press it down firmly, then twist to ensure the middle is cleanly cut out.

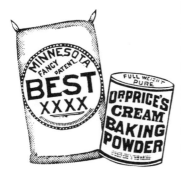

In an electric frying pan on medium/medium high heat, fry donuts and middles in oil until they are golden brown.

Shake warm donuts in bags filled with cinnamon sugar and/or powdered sugar. Leave some plain for diabetics.

PEPPERMINT PATTIES

A single recipe makes 64 patties or 2½ lbs.

Ingredients

1 14oz. can sweetened condensed milk
2 tsp. peppermint extract
12 drops red food coloring
1½–2 16oz. pkgs. confectioners sugar
1½ cups pecan halves

1. In large bowl, mix condensed milk, peppermint extract and food coloring. With spoon, stir in 1½ pkgs. confectioners sugar.

2. On cutting board(s) or table surface generously sprinkled with confectioners sugar, gradually knead in enough additional sugar so that mixture forms a smooth firm ball that doesn't stick to hands or table/board.

3. Pat mixture into 8" x 8" square. With a knife, cut it into 1" squares. Shape each piece into a ball and with fingers flatten into 2" patty-top with pecan half. Repeat with remaining pieces. Keep pieces covered with plastic wrap while preparing patties. Let patties dry 1 hour.

BAKED APPLES

5 apples, sliced in half and peeled
1 Tbsp butter
¼ cup sugar
pinch of cinnamon

Stir together cinnamon and sugar. Dip apple pieces in this mixture. Place butter in the baking dish and add apples. Cover with plastic and microwave on high for 7 to 9 minutes. Let stand 5 minutes before serving.

SNACKS

Engage residents in preparing simple finger foods such as carrot and celery sticks. Vegetable dips are easily prepared and look appetizing and colorful. Crackers and cheese and other snacks are also easy to prepare.

DESSERT

All you need for a tasty dessert is a pastry shell, a can of fruit and whipped cream. Have one resident whip the cream, while someone else pours the fruit into the pastry shell. The result is a mouth-watering sight to behold.

SALADS

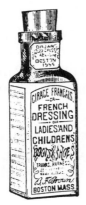

Residents can help prepare a cold chicken, fruit or salmon salad. Each person can carry out a particular step such as washing the vegetables and tossing the salad with dressing.

CHAPTER 8

Van Outings for Zero Cost

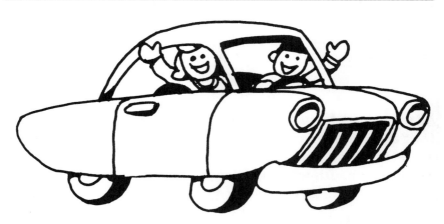

Going for a ride with residents is a very relaxing and pleasurable activity. They absolutely love it. If you aren't doing this already and have some form of transportation available, try scheduling rides bi-monthly, or even weekly. You will soon find it is a favorite activity.

There are many ways of wording "just driving around"—which is basically all you're doing, but how alluring does that sound? Here are some "motor-vating" suggestions for announcing outings:

EXPLORER'S CLUB

Explore new territory within the boundaries of the city. Has an old part of town been demolished and replaced with high-rises?

Are there any new buildings or major construction going on nearby that might be of interest to your passengers? It's always interesting to note how a city is changing or growing. Is there a new shopping mall in town? Is there a part of town residents are particularly curious about? Go a good distance and explore highlights of a neighboring town.

MYSTERY DRIVE

Make it an unknown destination. Of course, your mystery driver should know where you're going. Make it a short trip as some residents might not like the suspense. Have a guessing game on the way there. The person who guesses correctly gets to choose where the group will travel to next time.

BEACHCOMBERS CRUISE

If you are are lucky enough to be close to the beach, take a waterfront ride or a lake front drive. These are especially beautiful at sunrise and sunset. These drives are extremely popular if you don't mind the odd hours involved.

CITY TOUR

Divide your city in several sections and tour one each month. Focus on particular highlights that may be of special interest. Drive through a particularly fashionable residential section of beautiful homes. Daydream a bit. (Not the driver, please.)

41

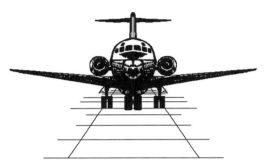

Airport Drive

Drive to an airport and watch the planes take off and land. The roof of a parking garage provides a particularly breathtaking view if accessible.

Tour Carvel Ice Cream

Carvel franchises often host group tours. Visitors learn how ice cream and other frozen treats are made. You will probably get a free sample at the end of the scheduled visit. (I have found the folks from Carvel to be very cooperative and helpful.)

Other Ideas for Outings:

Bakery

Call a favorite bakery in your vicinity and ask if they might give a tour or a cake-decorating demonstration for your group. Hopefully, they will let everyone try a little sample at the conclusion of your visit.

Donut Shop

It's fascinating to watch donuts being made, so try to schedule a tour to a donut shop. Warm donuts taste great too, incidentally.

Train Shop

An old fashioned train shop can hold residents' interest for quite some time, especially when the display trains are set to go when you get there. Arrange for someone to meet your group at the door and impart some interesting railroad facts.

BACK TO SCHOOL

Schedule a visit to a local preschool (preferably the school that regularly visits your residents). Have the director arrange for your residents to visit with the children in class.

ANTIQUE STORE

A trip to your local antique store will stimulate reminiscence and memory-making among residents. Try to find a store that has old farm implements and common household items from long ago. Let residents rifle through the objects and talk about their use.

CIRCUS

A trip to the circus will bring back happy childhood memories. Next time the circus comes to town, bring the residents along. Try to arrange a visit at a quiet time as large events like this can be too crowded.

SHOPPING

Take residents shopping. We tend to forget just how out of touch many residents are with today's prices. Show them foodstuff that was not available in their heyday (microwave packages). Talk to them about price changes over the years. Show them the new technology of scanning. Talk with them about the difference between the old General Store of long ago and today's supermarket.

CHAPTER 9

Unusual Party Ideas

There is nothing like a party to lift the spirits. Schedule regular parties for birthdays, anniversaries and holidays. Be flexible and don't shy away from holding an impromptu party when the situation calls for it. After lunch, after supper and before bed are good times for parties. Have a good line-up of musicians and entertainers that you can call in at short notice. Keep things simple. Avoid too much noise and excitement and have plenty of volunteers to help out. Make sure you have ample space for people to dance and move around. Serve a nice variety of snacks and beverages. Ready...get set...go.

Gay 90's

Have a special party to honor those residents 90 years of age and above. Make name tags to identify these special guests of honor and include their age (if there are no objections). Prizes could be awarded to the oldest residents and you could feature some guest speakers from the over 90 set. This could be a resident of the facility or some active retiree from your local community (they could speak on why they

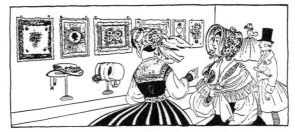

think they've lived so long). The possibilities are limitless.

For example, you could stage a show of music from the 1890's or early 1900's. Another fun thing to do might be to make a bulletin board of residents' baby or childhood pictures (without their names). Have a contest trying to guess who's who.

Veteran's Party

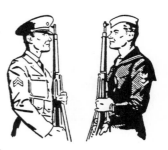

Call it what you will but set aside a date and time to hold a special event to honor Veterans of the World Wars. Experiment as you wish. You may decide to incorporate patriotic music into your program and perhaps have a retired military man speak to the group. Small pins can be made up with tiny American flags attached to identify those who have gone to war to preserve our country's honor. You could also try calling your local Veteran's Administration for more ideas.

Sandwich Party

Provide a table with ingredients and let residents create their own sandwiches. Incidentally, August is National Sandwich month.

National Doctor's Day

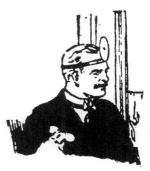

March 30 is National Doctor's Day and a great excuse for a party to honor your resident doctor(s). Make buttons for residents to wear that say "Thanks for Caring" or similar. In our facility, we put square tables together and served champagne for a toast to our house doctor. After the toast he gave a thank you speech. This was a nice intimate activity.

Tasting Parties

A tasting party makes a wonderful activity. Try some of these varieties or make up your own:

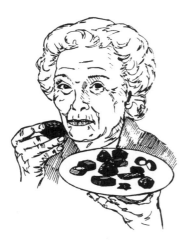

COFFEE TASTING

General Food International Coffees are easy to make (instant) and delicious as well. Some of the flavors include Irish Mint, Orange Cappuchino, Swiss Mocha and so on.

TEA TASTING

You'll find most interesting varieties in your grocery store. There are some wonderful herbal blends available.

POPCORN PARTY

Popcorn comes in many exotic flavors. Three old standbys include plain, caramel and cheese. Use your imagination.

HEALTH SNACKS

A health snack tasting party could be easily set up with the help of a local health food store. Yogurt-covered raisins or peanuts could be served. Ask the clerk about the difference between carob (chocolate substitute) and real chocolate. What are the benefits of these snacks? Jot down a few interesting facts about these tidbits to tell your guests at the party. You may even be able to get these things donated for the occasion. Find out if any of your residents' family members work at health food stores.

The tasting party theme is only limited to the power of your imagination. How about melon (water, canteloupe, honeydew and include other less-known varieties), cookie tasting (watch diabetics here), or even—dietetic snacks. Invite everyone to sample them.

The list goes on and on.

Pajama Party

For an enjoyable fun-packed evening, try a pajama party. Plan to have it in the early evening in two parts (make sure it's dark). Start off with the parade of the "pajama people" down the hallway through the main lobby. Offer prizes to participants wearing the funniest, prettiest or most colorful pajamas. The parade could end up in the living room with everyone being served hot chocolate. The music should be soft. Try playing lullabies or have someone read a bedtime story by candlelight. Again, use your imagination.

Cocktail Party

Almost everyone is staging cocktail parties these days. Vary the drink menu. For example, have a beer and pretzel party or serve ice cream drinks for a time. Any drink made with ice cream is smoother. Perhaps the kitchen can stretch the budget by contributing some vanilla ice cream. Good ice cream drinks are Grasshoppers, Pina Coladas, Kahlua Coladas, (coffee liquor in place of rum) Sombreros, Peaches and Cream (peach schnapps). If you are really intent on stretching your liquor budget or just lowering the alcohol content, there is always rum flavored extract to enhance the flavor that may be missing due to the frugality of the activity director.

Grandparents Bragging Party

You can't miss with this one! Invite all grandparents to bring pictures of their beloved grandchildren to the get-together. Honor the grandmother and grandfather with the most grandchildren, the youngest grandchild or whatever category you can think of. Since people love to talk about their families, this is a sure winner!

International Party Night

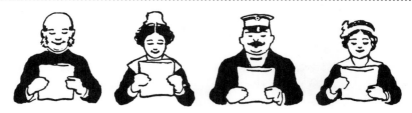

In St. Petersburg FL we are lucky to have the SPIFFS (St. Petersburg International Folk Fair Society) to help us out with this event. As is the case in many facilities, we have residents of different nationalities. When we have an international party, name tags which bear the color and symbols of each nationality are made. For example, the Irish wear shamrocks in green while the Italians have tiny replica Italian flags. The International Singers and Dancers put on an international fashion show of many different native costumes. If such a group is unavailable to you, ask families and friends of international residents to help by modeling things they might put together at home to represent different nations. A peasant blouse and full skirt or a Mexican dress would would work well. A Hawaiian outfit would create a festive air too.

Travel Party

If you can't find a travel agent to help you create a travel party, check your public library for travel-related films and plan the occasion around one particular geographic location. Ethnic themes are always good. Try arranging a Mexican, Spanish or French party (can can dancers would be a riot).

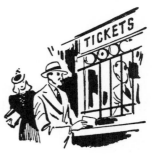

Perhaps your international residents and their families can be used as connections here.

These ideas work well:

HAWAIIAN

Use scenic posters from Hawaiian Week to decorate the room. A Hula girl wouldn't hurt the mood either. Serve Hawaiian punch and pineapple.

ITALIAN

Decorate the room with Italian flags. These can be made easily from construction paper. You can even serve a sheet cake decorated to resemble the Italian flag. It would be nice to feature Italian singers at this event. Check the local Italian/American Club for entertainer suggestions.

The party could be preceded by a spaghetti dinner and Italian ice cream. Try Spumone or Tortoni for dessert.

IRISH

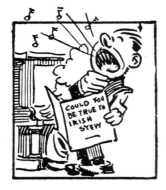

Everyone wears green, of course, for an Irish party and nothing works better than a sing-a-long. For a real crowd pleaser, try to find someone to do the Irish jig.

PATRIOTIC PARTY

Ideally a patriotic party is held in celebration of Independence Day, but it can be added to your yearly calendar at almost anytime. A patriotic sing-a-long is great entertainment and everyone can participate. Some residents may wish to get up and say a few words on behalf of our beloved country. Naturally, you will ask everyone to dress in red, white and blue.

For some cool refreshments, try this recipe instead of the usual cake. Scoop alternate layers of strawberry and vanilla ice cream to form a semi-pyramid on an aluminum foil covered serving tray. Buy small flags (on toothpicks or small plastic sticks) available in most stores and arrange them all over the pyramid.

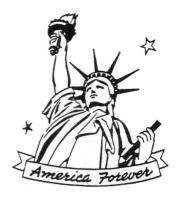

Just before serving, turn down the lights and place lighted sparklers in the mounds of ice cream. (Two will do fine). If possible, present your frozen, patriotic masterpiece to the tune of "Three Cheers for The Red, White and Blue." Soon after, there will be Three Cheers for You!

BASEBALL PARTY

Schedule a party around a locally televised ball game. Serve hot dogs, peanuts, cracker jacks or popcorn and don't forget the 7th inning stretch, an excellent time to slip in a few exercises. Play "Take Me Out To The Ballgame" sometime during this event, perhaps at the beginning to warm everyone up. Ask interested parties to take a guess at who will win the game and by how many points. Old timer baseball cards would be an ideal

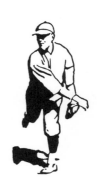

prize. Someone could recite "Casey At Bat" during a commercial break.

POSTCARD PARTY

Ask everyone to bring a postcard they have kept over the years. Award prizes for the oldest card (according to postmark), the most unusual or the prettiest. Give a prize for the card postmarked farthest away. You can even use a globe to show the distance!

ICE CREAM PARTY

Add even more flavor to ice cream socials by serving specialized frozen treats—banana split day, ice cream sodas, milkshakes, cones, sherbet party and so on. How about a sundae social where everyone makes his own sundae creations. Share this interesting fact—the ice cream cone was patented on September 22, 1903 by an Italian immigrant.

ANNIVERSARY PARTY

If your facility is lucky enough to house any married couples, don't forget to observe their wedding anniversaries! One terrific way to celebrate is to have them "get married again" as many couples do to renew their vows. If the couple agrees, everyone will have great fun dressing up the bride (don't forget the veil!) and groom for the ceremony. Borrow a top hat for the groom. This event could even be preceded by a surprise bridal shower for the lucky bride. Perfumes, scented soaps and maybe a (sexy) nightgown could be giv-

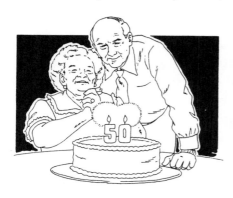

en. As a gag, scour the local thrift shops for a decent looking frying pan. Asking friends and employees of the facility for donations should result in some nice gifts (especially perfume and soap). Wrap all gifts in colorful paper and don't forget to sit the bride under an umbrella. It can be easily transformed into a bridal shower prop through your creative use of old lace scraps and crepe paper. Netting works well too.

Back to the wedding. Have a minister officiate (maybe someone whom everyone knows from regular Sunday services). Serve wedding cake. A white sheet cake appropriately decorated will do just fine. Is there someone in the facility family that has been recently married? Perhaps they can lend you the plastic bride and groom to adorn the cake? Ask. If not, use your imagination.

Last, but not least, the housekeeping department will kill you if you decide to throw rice. You must decide whether it is worth dying for. Take caution! Don't forget to put a "Just Married" sign on their door.

SINATRA PARTY

December 12 is Frank Sinatra's birthday. Since he was born in 1915, many of your residents will know his records well.

Show a Sinatra film (on your VCR) or play his old records. What do they remember about this heart throb of the 40s?

HALLOWEEN

Do you include children in your annual celebration of this ghoulish day? Hopefully so, because it makes the event much more fun.

Invite a local pre-school to bring their children, accompanied by their parents, for Halloween trick or treat night. Be sure to set up a definite time, say, from 6:30 till 8:00 P.M. Instead of letting little goblins run from room to room, set up several construction paper bats made by your craft class. At one station you could have a "pin the tail on the black cat" game. This may be made easily by tracing a Halloween decoration of black cat minus the tail, adding scary eyes and cutting several "tails" for partici-pants to pin on. No, of course you wouldn't use pins! Fold over some masking tape so it is sticky on all sides and place on back of the tail. Everyone wins at this game. Treats come after one attempt.

A haunted tunnel can be fashioned from two refrigerator-type boxes taped together. Spray paint it black and decorate accordingly. Hang spiders inside! Everyone who makes it through the tunnel gets a treat which leaves no one out. The games provide innocent fun and a good time for all. Let the residents coordinate the games and hand out candy. Encourage them to dress up for the fun of it! Most will.

When you contact the preschool ask the director to mention this idea to the parents. Undoubtedly, parents of young children these days will think this a great idea as many are afraid of letting their kids go trick or treating in the streets (who can blame them). Knowing this, they should be delighted with your invitation and you will have no problem whatsoever getting candy prize donations from these parents. After all, thanks to you the kids now have a chance to trick or treat and the parents won't have to worry.

Be sure to have a costume parade and award plenty of prizes for categories of your choice—the most original, funniest, scariest, prettiest costume. Have coffee on hand for the parents. They will hopefully be impressed and remember the name of your facility in times to come. (Not a bad way to get free publicity). Contact local newspapers and TV stations. They like to hear of these community events.

VALENTINE'S DAY PARTY

Although your first notion may be to recreate the scene of The St. Valentine's Day Massacre at your annual "V.D." party, please resist temptation and throw a nice little sweetheart ball or something safe like that. Valentine's day can be declared "Hug Day". Early that morning pin pink construction paper hearts with the words "Hug Me" on everybody. Start the trend yourself. It will soon become contagious. You can try asking residents to keep track of how many hugs they can give all day. Award the most frequent hugger with valentine candy, a heart shaped pillow or a similar prize.

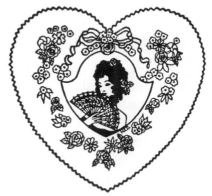

Decorations are easy to make for this one. Pink cake always goes down well too.

OCTOBERFEST

Don't leave this one out! Play German music (they have special Octoberfest records) and serve beer and pretzels. Only you will know that the beer isn't German, but anything that happens to be on sale that week. Is there a German American Club in your area to provide live entertainment? Perhaps some of your German descended residents have connections?

NEWSPAPER PARTY

Read through old newspapers in your library. Photocopy the famous headlines for each decade. Ask group members to bring a newspaper clipping to your meeting—the older the better. A most interesting party could consist of reading each entry as well as some of your own. This activity triggers reminiscing. You can even make a timeline of events headlined throughout the years. Prizes can be wrapped in newspaper.

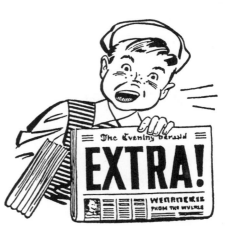

PIZZA PARTY

Going out for lunch is great, but of course, not everyone is able to go. Have pizzas delivered to your facility for an "Italian Pizza Party." Decorate the room with Italian flags which are easily made out of construction paper. As you enter the room, have a sign posted "Pizza Parlor" for all to see. Rolls of red checkered paper purchased at any party goods store make excellent tablecloths and can be thrown away after each use. Other "in house" luncheon party ideas may include a Chinese luncheon party or a fast food party (McDonald's?).

BEER & PRETZEL PARTY

Try serving the many pretzel variations found in your supermarket, as well as non-alcoholic beer. (Beer for thought!)

WINE AND CHEESE PARTY

You might wish to serve apple slices as well as crackers to accompany the wine and cheese.

STUFFED ANIMAL PARTY

Have your residents bring in their favorite stuffed animals. Award prizes to the oldest, the biggest or the silliest. Serve animal crackers. You may wish to do this in conjunction with the pajama party.

CHAPTER 10

Welcoming Activities

If you have a small group of ambulatory singers, they can greet new residents with a welcome song. Residents in wheelchairs can join in too. Select an easy tune that everyone knows, like *Twinkle Twinkle* or *Take Me Out to The Ballgame* and substitute your own words to suit the occasion. You may need a little help composing lyrics and if so, ask the residents to give assistance. Once you get something down you can use it time and time again until you have ambition enough to make up a new one. You might call your merry band of serenaders The Warbling Welcomers.

A welcoming committee can hold regular meetings and go about a variety of tasks. Members can volunteer as escorts when the occasions arise. An escort's main function is to personally invite and escort new (or more timid) residents to various functions. Try this and you may be pleasantly surprised to see attendance figures soar. People tend to be touched by and respond to a personal invitation. A personal invite says "you're important, you're wanted and your presence matters."

The welcoming committee can plan parties and put together little gifts to be presented to new "family members" on arrival. Appoint a public relations director and make it more official by presenting him with a badge stating his name and title.

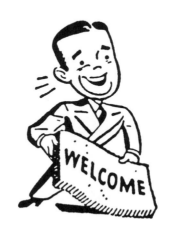

CHAPTER 11

Adult Education Programs

Colleges, community colleges and vocational schools in your area may have government grants on hand to conduct adult education classes in the community. Well, we're in the community right? Successful classes in long term care facilities include art appreciation, drawing for pleasure, American literature, United States history, bridge, world travel, music appreciation, earth science and many others. What a great way to spend what might be an otherwise boring evening. And what a great filler for your calender!

You need to do some research before getting this activity off the ground. Speak with residents and find out what their interests are. Go to your community college and find out what's available. Inquire if any facilities in your area have adult education programs in progress. If they have, pay them a visit. Ask questions. What programs have worked best? How are the classes funded? What has the resident response been?

Minicourses run by **The Institute of Lifelong Learning** introduce a variety of topics. A discussion leader's guide is available to assist those who want to organize and conduct a study group. To further assist discussion group leaders, the Institute designed two activity kits to correspond with minicourses produced in 1984 and '85. Kits contain supplemental material intended to enrich group study programs. **The Institute of Lifelong Learning** is a division of AARP and there is no charge for booklets or kits.

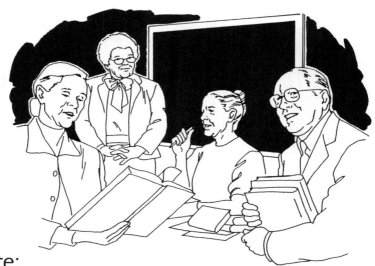

Write:

Minicourse
AARP Fulfillment
1909 K Street NW
Washington
DC 20049

CHAPTER 12

Fun With Books

Readers Club

For the bookworms among us, call the main branch of your public library and ask if they stock a good selection of large-print books. Inquire if they have a bookmobile unit that would drop books at your facility on a monthly basis. Many libraries now employ this outreach program with great success. If you are giving book reviews on your activities calendar, you may wish to select current library books. Appoint responsible residents as volunteer librarians with the promise that all librarians get first choice of incoming shipments. Most avid readers find this sufficient pay for lending a hand.

Poetry Reading

You may wish to initiate a poetry reading by picking a well-loved poet and reading from a collection of his famous works. Add your own special twist to this simple activity. Try reading by candlelight or outdoors (poems about nature). Save old greeting cards that contain particularly beautiful verses.

Book Making

Help residents make their own scrapbooks. Encourage them to cut interesting pictures from magazines relating to different topics. For example: food, weddings, children, Christmas, fashion, houses, travel or occupations. Help them cut out the pictures and paste them into a blank scrapbook. They will take pride in having made the book and will get many hours of quiet pleasure from leafing through its contents.

Read and Reminisce

Find a color picture book about the old days and share its contents with residents. This works well as a bedside activity. Time Life Books has a wonderful series called **This Fabulous Century**. Each book is devoted to a particular decade and describes in words and pictures the fads, the music, politics and major events of the decade. You will find these books (which are now out of print) and others like them in used book stores and thrift stores.

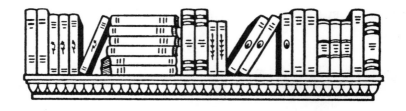

CHAPTER 13

A Laugh a Minute— Comedy Hour

There is currently much interest in the therapeutic benefits of humor. We all know that we feel better after a hearty laugh, but did you know that laughter sets off the physiological processes that help make us feel better? Laughing releases endorphins into the brain. As a result, a natural high is created (similar to the effect of various mood-altering drugs) and stress and tension are released.

Put this magical approach to work in your activities program by scheduling a comedy hour. Show videotapes of old comedies by the Marx brothers, Lucille Ball and Charlie Chaplin to get the laughter juices flowing. Find out when old radio comedy shows are being repeated and tape them for residents.

Get a good book of jokes from the library and read excerpts from books of humor. Reader's Digest provides great humorous material which can be used to entertain residents. Arrange chairs in a circle while telling jokes. Once you get started you will more than likely jog the memory of others who will want to tell their share of jokes as well. HA!

CHAPTER 14

Keeping Fit

Since nursing home residents are inclined to lead sedentary lives, exercise becomes all-important. Among its many benefits, exercise helps people sleep better at night. It is also enjoyable, helps to relieve tension and anxiety and generally lifts the spirits. Following are ideas for active games to help your residents stay in shape.

Bowling

Bowling is enjoyable and provides good exercise. There are many light and inexpensive bowling sets available in sport shops and from mail order companies. Set ten bowling pins up in a triangular configuration. You should have four rows of one, two, three and four pins. Even wheelchair bound residents will be able to take a shot at knocking the pins over. Each success is greeted with a loud and enthusiastic cheer.

Walking Races

Hold a walking race for ambulatory residents. Enlist the help of volunteers to escort residents and set the pace. Wait for the cheers as people approach the finishing line. You can also hold races for wheelchair-bound residents. Space, organization and plenty of help are absolute essentials for this activity.

Beanbag Toss

Beanbags are popular with older residents. They are also light and easy to handle. Have residents toss their bean bags into a basket. Give a point for each hit.

Balloon Toss

Balloons are colorful and easy to handle. They have pleasant associations for most people. Seat players in a circle. Give each one a colored bat and have them bat the ball around the circle. This game can last much longer than you might anticipate as people tend to get immersed in it and lose track of time.

Darts

Playing darts can be fun and safe. Avoid using darts with steel points. There are many sets now available with suction cups. When they hit the metal target, they stick to it. Velcro dart boards with velcro-covered balls are also widely available at toy stores now.

Parachute Toss

If you haven't got access to a parachute (not many people do!), use an old sheet as a substitute. Tossing the 'parachute' is an ideal group activity and excellent for exercise and using hand and eye coordination. Players grab the edges of the sheet. Balloons and balls are tossed into the center and the players toss them around. The objective is to keep them moving and not let them fall off the sheet. This activity is ideal for residents who are wheelchair-bound.

Shuffleboard

Small wooden disks are pushed with a shuffleboard stick as far as they will go on the shuffleboard base. The game is easy to play, it provides good exercise and the equipment can be made at little cost.

Volleyball

String up a net and place chairs on either side. Now you have created two teams. The beachball is tossed back and forth across the net. Balloons can also be used.

Indoor Badminton

Indoor badmiton is another fun activity. Arrange it the same way as balloon volleyball so that residents are seated on both sides of the net.

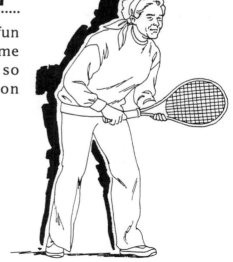

CHAPTER 15

Animal Love: Pet Therapy

Pet therapy is a great concept that really works. Animals are not prejudiced against the elderly community (as people sometimes are). They look for love and affection from residents and are well able to reciprocate. Therapeutic touch is exceptionally important. Many residents are simply starved for a loving handclasp, a hug or gentle embrace. When nursing home residents are allowed free contact with animals, the benefits of this interchange are readily visible. One need only provide the setting and sit back to enjoy as the room is warmed by love.

Taking in a pet on a full-time basis may be a great idea but there are some considerations that apply. Will the pet be indoors or out? Where will it sleep when the climate gets cold. Siberian Huskies are built to weather icy conditions but most canines get cold when left outside. Who will take responsibility for the animal? Most of the time able residents will volunteer to share in the care and feeding of your family pet, but ultimately the responsibility rests with the activity director. Be sure to check out what that entails.

Dog Day Afternoons

Weekly visits from furry friends may be the best idea of all. One day a week can be scheduled as Dog Day with area volunteers supplying pets to be adopted for an hour or two that day. Call the SPCA or Humane Society. Inquire also as to whether any residents have families or friends who might wish to participate in the program. Be cautious of this route though as some residents can feel jealous of family pets giving attention to others. Or, bring your own pet.

Birds on Wheels

If your facility has a canary or parakeet in a cage, wheel it around to different parts of the facility and to individual rooms. These birds make very lively and entertaining pets. You could also consider setting up an aviary outside with such birds as parakeets, cockatiels and budgerigars.

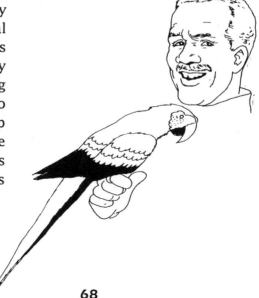

Fish

Fish are wonderful company. Colorful and quiet, they help to brighten up the surroundings. Recent research has shown that watching fish is relaxing, that blood pressure and heart rate are reduced as a result and that they produce a calming effect. They are also easy to look after. Make sure your facility has an aquarium and encourage residents to walk over daily and talk to the fish.

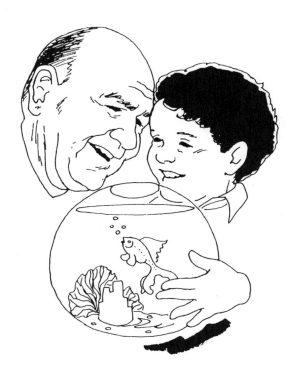

CHAPTER 16

Special Shows

Floral Arranging Demonstrations

These demonstrations can easily be arranged through your local florist. If you do a lot of business with one particular florist, all the better! Have a drawing of all those present and award the finished centerpiece to one lucky winner.

Vacation by Imagination

Invite someone to come in and show their vacation slides, pictures and souvenirs as well as artifacts from their own trip. The more exotic or faraway the destination, the better. Serve refreshments to complement the theme.

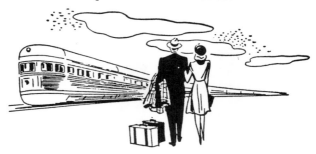

Antique Car Show

Plan this full-day activity on a Saturday or Sunday. Try contacting local antique auto clubs. All the better if you know someone involved in such an organization. They work hard to make their cars look beautiful and they love to show them off. Rope off an area. If you have your own parking lot and can be assured there will be no other traffic, you're in business! Ask if car-owners wouldn't mind rounding out the

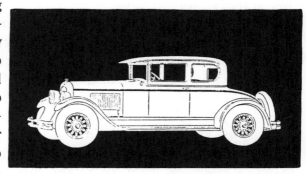

day by offering rides to your residents. Take plenty of pictures. Set up an old fashioned lemonade stand to refresh your visitors. You may or may not wish to invite the public, but certainly invite your residents' relatives. Think about inviting your local press or TV station.

Hat Day

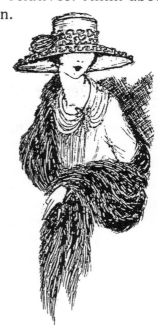

Designate one day on your calendar as **Hat Day**. Have an antique or unusual hat display set up in the morning featuring a variety of interesting toppers obtained from different sources. An afternoon hat parade should feature residents and staff alike on a promenade through the main hallways and lobby wearing an assortment of hats for all to admire. Follow up the parade with a **Mad Hatters Tea Party**. Here, each person must must wear a hat for admission. Award prizes for the biggest hat, the silliest or the prettiest. Anyone who can do the Mexican hat dance could also add amusement to the day!

Glamor day for the ladies

Find an ambitious Avon lady to lend profitable assistance to this activity. Set up several display tables to include perfume, lipstick, jewelry, etc. One table may include wine,

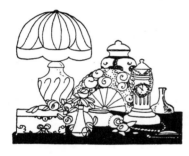

cheese and crackers to be enjoyed by glamorous guests. Invite ladies to a "makeover" and have mirrors on hand so they can enjoy the transformation. If Avon is currently having a sale, advertise it in poster size so interested residents can take advantage. Encourage them to try new shades or eye makeup if they have never worn it. The whole idea is to try to make them feel good about themselves. To boost sales, include the staff.

Exotic Plant Show

Call a local nursery (preferably in their slow season) and ask if they would allow an employee to come to your facility to set up a plant display. The more unusual or striking plants are most attractive. Write the names of plants in large black letters on index cards along with any interesting facts and how to care for them. While it should not be billed as a plant sale, many residents (or employees) may wish to purchase greenery for their rooms. Jot individual prices down on the backs of the index cards. The nursery employee will almost certainly go back to the garden center with a lighter load and this should be mentioned to the manager when initially trying to set up the event.

Antique Show

Another fascinating display is one of antiques. Contact an antique dealer and ask to borrow some items for display. Choose things that residents may remember from their youth. This activity will inspire conversation about "the good old days."

CHAPTER 17

Christmas Celebrations

This time of year usually takes care of itself on the activities agenda.

In general, people feel more charitable around the Christmas season so do take advantage of those who wish to volunteer their services at this time. Schedule church and school choirs as well as old fashioned carolers as often as possible. Groups like these usually look for places to bring the Christmas message. Don't play hard to get. Dredge up that old phone book and call them. Ask them to keep you in mind for any other productions or special services they may have throughout the year.

Scenic Drive

A Christmas-time scenic drive is magical. Take them on a "nighttime fantasy" drive to see well-lit houses and businesses in your area. One sure bet for a sparkling holiday ride is to take a drive past several local florist shops. They always outdo themselves with decorative lights and other such seasonal attractions.

Breakfast with Santa

Reserve a special room (such as the activities or card room) and use an electric skillet to make a special breakfast with Santa. Serve French toast or Blueberry pancakes. Coordinate the remainder of the meal with the kitchen staff. Your menu could read something like this:

Jingle Berry Juice (cranberry juice)

Festive French Toast

Fresh Fruit in Season

Coffee/Milk

Decorate a special chair for your guest of honor. Play "Here Comes Santa Clause" on the record player for his grand entrance. If you can find a talented Santa to play a tune on the piano or tell a few jokes, all the better! Invite residents to have their pictures taken with him. After displaying them on your bulletin board for all to see, give them out to individuals as keepsakes.

A Trip To The North Pole

A "Trip to the North Pole To Visit Santa" is bound to bring about some chuckles. Print the announcement in the newsletter and it will surely stir up considerable curiosity. Here's the good news. You don't actually have to drive all that way just to see Saint Nick. (I know you're relieved). Just arrange to take residents to a local mall for a short chat and a group picture with Santa. Be sure to post that picture on a bulletin board for all to see. Folks visiting the facility will get a kick out of this, too.

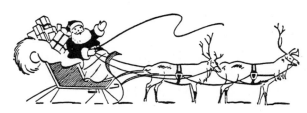

Christmas Van

Do you have a company van or station wagon for transportation? If so, why not make it a group project to decorate it for Christmas. One suggestion is to wrap it in ribbon just like a giant Christmas package (as seen on several florist trucks). Don't forget the bow on top! Stretch bright red or green shelf paper across and down the vehicle. Skip over the windshield or you will impair the driver's vision. Party good stores offer more heavy duty materials that can be used as ribbon. Life size pictures of Santa and his helpers can be fastened to inside windows on the side of the vehicle to imply that they are actual passengers. Draw waving hands in appropriate sizes so it looks like your unusual passengers are waving to passersby. If the name of your facility is printed on the outside, all the better! What a wonderful advertisement on wheels!

Carol Sing-A-Long

Do you have a carol sing-a-long on your December calendar? For a little spice, ask a resident possessing a gifted voice to lead it.

In St. Petersburg, Florida, where we are lucky enough to experience lovely holiday weather, we staged an outdoor "carol by candlelight" party in our beautifully decorated courtyard. Outdoor candles line the courtyard adding a perfect romantic glow to the occasion. We made candles by filling paper bags (lunch size) with sand deep enough to hold a utility candle, about four inches. The sand also protects against danger in case the bag should blow over. Fold the top of the bag down about two cuffs and the effect is enchanting! A strolling accordionist wandered about the courtyard playing the melodies of Christmas. A perfect evening! (We did it Christmas Eve!)

Bus-Caroling

If there is a vehicle at your disposal, why not take the group caroling in the bus! Make tapes of well-known Christmas songs to play during the ride. Have residents join in singing Jingle Bells out open windows, weather permitting. (We are lucky here in Florida!) Make strategic stops in driveways to sing to a chosen few. We pulled off one such feat by showing up in the driveway of our administrator (all decked out in Santa caps!) singing "We Wish You A Merry Christmas"

Chanukah

Even if your facility can boast of only one Jewish resident, you simply must in some way observe this festival of lights holiday occasion. Although this is the highlight of the year for those with Hebrew heritage it can be made a fun and informative celebration for everyone. Contact a temple to obtain information about local Jewish organizations who might be of assistance in planning a Chanukah program at your facility. That should get things underway. If there is a Jewish community center in your city, ask if children can come visit.

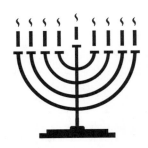

Appendix

BOOKS FOR ACTIVITY DIRECTORS

Free Things For Activity Directors
by Debra Cassistre

This revised and expanded edition of Debra Cassistre's book lists hundreds of items that can be obtained free—including books, games, posters, movies and craft items. It's message is clear and simple: activity directors can create a quality program with exciting resources even if they are on a tight budget. $10.95

Failure-Free Activities for the Alzheimer's Patient
by Carmel Sheridan

This award-winning book describes hundreds of simple, non-threatening activities which are suitable for persons with Alzheimer's disease. The author describes how to focus on the abilities that remain rather than the patient's deficits and shows how to create activities which capitalize on existing strengths. $10.95

Reminiscence:
Uncovering A Lifetime of Memories
by Carmel Sheridan

Reminiscing is one of the most powerful healing activities for people with Alzheimer's disease. This book explains the simple techniques involved in stimulating memories. It outlines themes to explore as well as hundreds of meaningful activities involving reminiscence. $12.95

Index

Order Form

Send To:
Elder Books PO Box 490   Forest Knolls CA 94933
415 488-9002 or FAX to 415 488-4720

Please send me:

___ Copies of Activity Ideas for the Budget Minded @ $10.95

___ Copies of Free Things for Activity Directors @ $10.95

___ Copies of Failure-Free Activities @ $10.95

___ Copies of Reminiscence @ $12.95

SHIPPING: $2.75 for first book, $1.75 for each additional book.
CA residents, please add 8.25% sales tax.

Total for books..$_____.___

Total sales tax ....$_____.___

Total shipping..$_____.___

Amount enclosed ....$_____.___

Name _____

Address: _____

City: _____ State: ___ Zip: _____

☐ CHECK HERE FOR FREE CATALOG